National Audit Office

AF885311

Report
by the Comptroller
and Auditor General

Department for Work & Pensions

The Work Programme

HC 266 SESSION 2014-15 2 JULY 2014

Our vision is to help the nation spend wisely.

Our public audit perspective helps Parliament hold government to account and improve public services.

The National Audit Office scrutinises public spending for Parliament and is independent of government. The Comptroller and Auditor General (C&AG), Amyas Morse, is an Officer of the House of Commons and leads the NAO, which employs some 820 employees. The C&AG certifies the accounts of all government departments and many other public sector bodies. He has statutory authority to examine and report to Parliament on whether departments and the bodies they fund have used their resources efficiently, effectively, and with economy. Our studies evaluate the value for money of public spending, nationally and locally. Our recommendations and reports on good practice help government improve public services, and our work led to audited savings of £1.1 billion in 2013.

National Audit Office

Department for Work & Pensions

The Work Programme

Report by the Comptroller and Auditor General

Ordered by the House of Commons
to be printed on 1 July 2014

This report has been prepared under Section 6 of the National Audit Act 1983 for presentation to the House of Commons in accordance with Section 9 of the Act

Amyas Morse
Comptroller and Auditor General
National Audit Office

30 June 2014

HC 266 | £10.00

This report compares performance of the Work Programme to previous welfare-to-work programmes and the Department's aims.

10472 07/14 NAO

Contents

The National Audit Office study team consisted of:
Terry Caulfield, Rebecca Sidell and Andrew Tuffin, under the direction of Max Tse

This report can be found on the National Audit Office website at www.nao.org.uk

For further information about the National Audit Office please contact:

National Audit Office
Press Office
157–197 Buckingham Palace Road
Victoria
London
SW1W 9SP

Tel: 020 7798 7400

Enquiries: www.nao.org.uk/contact-us

Website: www.nao.org.uk

Twitter: @NAOorguk

Key facts

£2.8bn	2.1m	£450m
Department's forecast – total payments to prime contractors, June 2011 to March 2020	Department's forecast – referrals to the Work Programme, June 2011 to March 2016	Department's forecast – total savings to benefit spending from the Work Programme compared to the baseline agreed with HM Treasury

296,000	people secured job outcomes up to March 2014
£41 million	saving on the amount the Department would have spent between June 2011 and March 2020 for similar levels of performance on previous welfare-to-work programmes
212	minimum service standards that prime contractors proposed in their bids
£11 million	estimated cost of sustainment payments up to March 2014 where the Department cannot confirm employment
£21 million	saved by the Department by extrapolating invalid job outcome payments and reducing payments to prime contractors accordingly
£31 million	likely total cost in 2014-15 of incentive payments to prime contractors to reward high performance

Summary

1 The Department for Work & Pensions (the Department) is responsible for the Work Programme, the government's scheme to help long-term unemployed people to find and keep jobs. The Department expects to refer 2.1 million people to the Work Programme between June 2011 and March 2016, at a total cost of £2.8 billion.

2 The Work Programme aims to increase employment, and reduce the time that people spend on benefits. In particular it aims to improve support for those who are harder-to-help. The Department expected to achieve these aims for a lower cost per referral than previous welfare-to-work initiatives.

3 The Department refers people to the Work Programme, usually after they have been unemployed for between 9 and 12 months. The Department assigns people to different payment groups depending on factors such as age or benefit type. In this report we distinguish between easier-to-help groups such as Jobseeker's Allowance claimants and harder-to-help groups such as people who claim Employment and Support Allowance.[1]

4 The Department pays prime contractors to provide support using a payment-by-results approach. The amount each prime contractor receives depends largely on its success in getting people into sustained work. The Department pays a different amount depending on the participant's payment group.

5 Contractors can be private, public or third sector organisations. Prime contractors choose how to support people, such as subcontracting some or all of the support. The Department maintains 40 contracts in 18 different geographic areas across England, Wales, and Scotland. Each area has at least two prime contractors and the Department refers people randomly between contractors in their local area. Currently there are 18 different prime contractors and around 700 subcontractors.

6 The Department will stop referring people to the Work Programme after March 2016. Payments under current contracts will continue for a further four years. The Department is looking at a range of options for its welfare-to-work provision from April 2016.

1 Our distinction is a relative one as most people referred to the Work Programme have been out of work for a long period and could be seen as hard-to-help. We also recognise that payment groups do not match directly to how hard individual people are to help, particularly for smaller payment groups such as Employment and Support Allowance volunteers. For the purposes of this report we refer primarily to Jobseeker's Allowance 18 to 24 (payment group 1) and Jobseeker's Allowance 25 and over (payment group 2) as examples of easier-to-help groups, and new Employment and Support Allowance claimants (payment group 6) as harder-to-help.

Scope of this report

7 This is our third report on the Work Programme. In January 2012, we reported on the Work Programme's design and introduction. In December 2012 we summarised the Department's first set of published performance data. The Committee of Public Accounts has published two reports on the Work Programme after taking evidence from the Department.

8 In this report we consider the value for money of the Work Programme. We review performance up to March 2014 and consider the Department's:

- aims for the Work Programme (Part One);
- performance for easier-to-help groups (Part Two);
- performance for harder-to-help groups (Part Three); and
- control of the Work Programme's costs (Part Four).

9 The Department designed the Work Programme to improve on previous welfare-to-work programmes. We therefore compare performance to previous programmes as a first test of value for money. The Department also had expectations about how the Work Programme would work and how much it would improve performance; we also compare performance against this more challenging benchmark. Figure 21 in Appendix One summarises this approach.

10 Performance comparisons are inherently difficult without a clear control group. The effectiveness of welfare-to-work support is determined by its additional impact on employment compared to what would have happened without support. But baseline performance is uncertain and could change over time. Comparisons with other programmes are also affected by differences in scheme design, performance measurement and economic conditions. We make judgements based on the available evidence, and we discuss limitations in Appendix Three.

Key findings

Performance for easier-to-help payment groups

11 The Work Programme has helped people claiming Jobseeker's Allowance who have completed two years get into and stay in work at about the same rate as previous welfare-to-work schemes. Performance in getting people into work has improved since the first published data. Of those people claiming Jobseeker's Allowance aged 25 and over, 27 per cent have moved into employment lasting six months or longer. This is similar to previous comparable programmes. People are also sustaining employment at about the same level as in previous programmes, with younger claimants sustaining work more than expected (paragraphs 2.3 to 2.5; 2.10 and 2.11).

12 This performance has not so far achieved the Department's higher expectations, but it expects recent improvements to continue. The most recent monthly cohort to have completed the programme achieved job outcomes for 32 per cent of participants. This is below the Department's original forecast (39 per cent) and bidders' original expectations (42 per cent), but approaching minimum performance levels (33 per cent). The Department expects that performance will continue to improve for remaining cohorts based on the early performance of more recent cohorts still in the programme. The Department expects a significant improvement with Jobseeker's Allowance claimants aged 25 and over achieving job outcomes in 38 per cent of referrals. If sustained this would be a material improvement on preceding programmes.

13 Recent analysis by the Department suggests that many job outcomes are not claimed by contractors. The Department has used HM Revenue & Customs' data to estimate that contractors have not claimed job outcomes for around 26,000 people who did get into work for the required length of time. Up to March 2014 there were 296,000 outcomes across all payment groups and cohorts so the Department's estimate would increase measured performance by around 9 per cent. We have not validated the data supporting the Department's estimate and it is not clear how much previous programmes were also affected by under-reporting (paragraphs 2.12 to 2.14).

14 Jobseeker's Allowance claimants are spending less time on benefits than the Department expected. While employment outcomes are similar, the Department expects the Work Programme to reduce peoples' average time on benefit compared with previous welfare-to-work schemes. The Department does not know why participants are spending less time on benefit, although this is consistent with contractors under-claiming outcomes. The Department expects to save £450 million in total across all payment groups between June 2011 and March 2020 compared to the baseline agreed with HM Treasury (paragraphs 2.15 and 2.16).

Performance for harder to help payment groups

15 The Department set initial performance expectations too high. The initial performance expectation and minimum performance level for Employment and Support Allowance claimants was that 22 per cent of people would achieve a job outcome. The Department accepts this level was set too high. Since November 2012 the Department has also referred Employment and Support Allowance claimants with a 12 month prognosis before being ready for work. These people are less likely to find work and performance is pulled down by the change in the mix of referrals. The Department has revised its expectations of performance downwards (paragraphs 3.3 and 3.4).

16 Performance for harder-to-help groups is still below expectations and about the same as previous programmes, but the Department expects further improvements. The Department designed the Work Programme to help participants who face significant barriers to employment. Performance for Employment and Support Allowance claimants who have completed the programme (11 per cent) is still below expectations (22 per cent) and previous programmes (12 per cent). But performance has improved from the very low levels at the start of the programme and early performance of more recent cohorts is showing signs of further improvement (paragraph 3.5).

17 On average, prime contractors have reduced what they plan to spend on the hardest-to-help. The support for the Work Programme's harder-to-help participants is lower than for those with better employment prospects. Providers' own estimates show that they plan to spend 54 per cent less on each participant in harder-to-help groups than when they bid. Several contractors told us that they do not use payment groups to help target support, and that funding for harder-to-help groups is lower than expected (paragraphs 3.7 and 3.9).

18 The Department has had to change its approach to maintaining minimum levels of service. The Department intended that minimum service standards would help to guarantee the quality of service received by all participants regardless of their barriers to employment. The Department originally allowed contractors to set their own minimum service standards. Contractors set 212 standards and the Department could not monitor these effectively. In July 2013, the Department introduced a new monitoring regime but the Department has limited ability to identify issues such as parking of harder-to-help participants (paragraphs 3.10 to 3.14).

Controlling costs

19 The Work Programme has reduced risks to the Department of paying for low performance. It expected to pay contractors £1.7 billion between June 2011 and March 2014. Because performance was lower than it expected in the first year of the Work Programme the Department actually paid £1.4 billion. It is difficult to make direct comparisons with previous programmes but for roughly similar levels of performance the Department is paying around £41 million (2 per cent) less for the Work Programme than it would have done for previous schemes (paragraphs 4.2 and 4.3).

20 Contractors expect lower profits as a result of lower performance and referrals. Overall contractors still expect to make a profit on the Work Programme although the amount they most recently forecast is 57 per cent lower than when they bid. The contractor market appears to be sustainable. No prime contractor has left the Work Programme since the Department introduced it in June 2011, although there have been a number of takeovers and mergers. Contractors have raised concerns about the Work Programme's viability and in some cases were seeking out other sources of work to supplement the Work Programme. The Department has not monitored contractors' profits under previous welfare-to-work programmes (paragraphs 4.4 to 4.8).

21 The Department has improved its validation of job outcome payments. The Department checks job outcome claims and extrapolates rates of invalid claims to reduce payments to contractors. The Department estimates that its approach has saved it £21 million up to March 2014. The validation regime may also have deterred contractors from claiming some outcomes. It continues to improve its approach. For example, it has removed requirements to get permission before contacting employers and has learnt how to elicit more accurate information about employment (paragraph 4.10 to 4.12).

22 **The Department is still paying prime contractors for potentially invalid sustainment payments.** Although the overall cost of the Work Programme is lower than previous programmes, the Department may be paying contractors for performance they are not actually achieving. The Department estimates how many claims for sustainment payments might be invalid, but it does not extrapolate its estimate and claw back a proportion of payments. As a result, the Department estimates that it has incurred losses of £11 million to March 2014. The Department is taking steps to improve validation. Without changing its approach the Department might otherwise pay a further £25 million over the remaining programme for potentially invalid claims (paragraphs 4.13 to 4.18).

23 **Flawed contractual performance measures mean the Department will have to make incentive payments to even the worst performing contractors.** The Department established incentive payments to reward high performance. But it uses a measure of performance that is highly sensitive to changes in referral volumes over time. In 2014-15 all 40 contracts are likely to be entitled to £31 million in incentive payments. The Department estimates that only £6 million would be paid using an accurate measure of performance (paragraph 4.21).

24 **Contractual performance measures have also made it more expensive to terminate contracts of poor performing contractors.** Following a review of contracts, the Department has issued a notice of termination to one contract held by the Newcastle College Group. Because the contractor had not technically breached the performance measures in the contract, the Department issued the notice under a voluntary break clause and not for any breach of contract. The Department is negotiating termination costs with the contractor (paragraphs 4.23 to 4.24).

25 **The Department has changed contracts several times to address limitations in the original contracts.** The Department introduced the Work Programme quickly in 2011, when payment-by-results was a new approach. The Department recognised the need to adapt contracts and introduced over 30 contract variations with contractors. It estimates that changes have avoided increased costs of around £40 million over the life of the programme (paragraphs 4.25 and 4.26).

Conclusion on value for money

26 After a poor start, the performance of the Work Programme is at similar levels to previous programmes. Current published data may understate actual job outcomes and the Department is also forecasting further improvements over the rest of the programme. At the same time the Department has reduced costs and reduced the risks of paying for poor performance. There are positive signs that the Work Programme has improved on previous welfare-to-work programmes and has the potential to offer value for money, particularly if the Department can achieve the much higher rates of performance that it now expects for the remainder of the programme.

27 It is not yet clear that the Work Programme has substantially improved on past performance or met its other aims for helping people into work. In particular the Department has struggled to improve outcomes for harder-to-help groups. Contrary to the intentions of the Work Programme, contractors are spending less on people in these groups and there are signs that some people receive very little support. The Work Programme is also not working as the Department intended in the way it rewards contractors for performance. Flaws in contracts and performance measures have led to unnecessary and avoidable costs.

28 To demonstrate that the Work Programme offers value for money, the Department will need to show that it can build on recent improvements and deliver actual results to match the significant and sustained increases in performance it now expects. The Department has recognised it also needs to make changes to contracts and performance measures and reduce unnecessary payments.

29 The Department has not cleared the findings in this report on the grounds that they do not reflect the Department's view of the relevant facts.

Recommendations

30 The Department recognises the need to improve performance and address issues we have raised. In developing the Work Programme and future contracted out welfare-to-work schemes it should:

a **Ensure sufficient time to develop a robust performance framework**

- The Department should avoid rolling out future programmes before it has had time to develop contracts and the performance framework.
- It should assume that, like the Flexible New Deal and the Work Programme, future programmes may have slow starts and uncertain volumes and factor this into decisions about timing, roll-out and design.
- The Department should identify ways to assess contractors' additional impact on participants' employment outcomes using control groups.

b **Improve the setting and monitoring of minimum service standards**

- The Department should review any findings from post-Work Programme evaluation and views on how the Work Programme has affected the prospects for people who complete two years on the programme without finding a job.
- The Department should review whether payment groups require different minimum service standards, for example, where particular barriers to work exist.
- Even where minimum standards are common across payment groups, the Department should monitor minimum service standards by payment group, rather than just overall, to ensure that contractors are not 'parking' people.
- The Department should gather other standard measures of services (beyond minimum service levels) in order to identify good practice or potential 'parking'.

c **Eliminate spending on invalid sustainment payments**

- The Department is negotiating with contractors over a new approach to sustainment payments and will need to show it has eliminated invalid payments to contractors.
- It should set out: how much contractors have returned from past payments; the new arrangements for sustainment payments; and the costs the Department has incurred to agree new contracts, for example by increasing payment levels.
- In future programmes the Department should review contracts to identify whether similar problems might arise.

d **Improve performance management measures**

- Providers should not receive incentive payments based on flawed measures of performance. The Department recognises that minimum performance levels have not worked well in managing contracts and has developed a new cohort-based measure of performance.
- Future programmes should use cohort-based measures for determining whether an incentive payment is merited, introduce relative as well as absolute thresholds, or remove these payments altogether.
- The Department should extend its use of the HM Revenue & Customs' real-time information to help prime contractors to identify people that are no longer in employment to support them back into work.

e **Develop a clear approach to making any future termination decisions**

- After it has agreed termination costs, the Department should evaluate the impact of terminating a contract.
- It should set out clear principles for making future termination decisions using break clauses in the current contracts.
- In future contracts it should include relative as well as better absolute measures of performance in setting the conditions under which it could terminate contracts at no cost.

Part One

Aims of the Work Programme

1.1 The Department introduced the Work Programme in June 2011 to help long-term unemployed people get and keep jobs. In this part we look at the Work Programme's:

- aims;
- differences from previous programmes; and
- development over time.

Improving on previous welfare-to-work programmes

1.2 The Department introduced the Work Programme because it considered existing welfare-to-work programmes had performed poorly. The Department considered that both Pathways to Work and Flexible New Deal had 'failed to live up to expectations'[2] and it set four aims for improvement (**Figure 1**).

Figure 1
Work Programme's aims

The Department established four aims compared to previous welfare-to-work programmes

Aims	Measuring success
Move more participants into work	An increase in the rate at which participants move into sustained employment
Move participants into work sooner	A decrease in the average time participants are on benefit
Move participants into work for longer	An increase in average time in employment for a participant
Lead to less 'parking' of harder-to-help groups	A reduction in the gap between off flow/time in employment rates for disadvantaged groups compared to other participants

Source: Department for Work & Pensions' *Outline Business Case*, November 2010

2 Department for Work & Pensions' Outline Business Case, November 2010.

1.3 As on previous welfare-to-work programmes, the Department refers people to prime contractors for support. Compared with past programmes the Department aimed to encourage innovation and performance by:

- giving contractors longer to work with participants and more flexibility to decide how to support them;
- improving incentives for contractors to achieve sustained outcomes and to support harder-to-help groups; and
- developing competition between contractors to improve performance.

More flexibility for contractors

1.4 The Work Programme addresses concerns about previous welfare-to-work programmes by giving support for longer. The Department refers people to the Work Programme when they have been unemployed for a time ranging from immediately to 12 months depending on the benefit a person claims. People then stay on the Work Programme for two years (**Figure 2** overleaf). By comparison, contractors for Flexible New Deal had one year to work with participants.

1.5 Contractors also have more flexibility in how they support people. The Department refers people to prime contractors who decide how to support people. Prime contractors may work with people directly, or may refer them to specialist subcontractors.

Improving incentives for sustained employment

1.6 In previous programmes the Department paid contractors for specific forms of support as well as for job outcomes. For example, under Flexible New Deal 60 per cent of actual payments were outcome based. The Work Programme relies much more heavily on payment-by-results, and the Department expects 80 per cent of payments to be outcome based. Contractors can claim:

- **An attachment payment** for taking a participant on to the Work Programme. This is a fixed payment and reduces to nil in 2014-15.
- **A job outcome payment** when a participant has been in work for a cumulative period, such as three or six months.
- **A sustainment payment** for every four weeks someone is in work beyond the job outcome period.

Figure 2
Overview of the Work Programme

The Department refers people to contractors for support over a two year period

	Description	Timing for a Jobseeker's Allowance 25 and over
Referral	**Jobcentre Plus** refers **participants** to a randomly chosen **prime contractor** in their area	After 12 months unemployment
Attachment	The **prime contractor** registers attachments for **participants** **Participants** receive support from the **prime contractor**	Within 15 days of referral
Off benefit	**Participants** stop claiming benefits resulting in a saving to government	Any time after attachment
Job outcome achieved	A **participant** achieves six months of cumulative employment **Department** pays **prime contractors** for confirmed job outcomes	From 6 to 30 months after attachment
Sustainment achieved	**Prime contractors** receive a payment for each month of further employment a **participant** achieves	From 7 to 43 months after attachment
Completed programme without an outcome	Unemployed **participants** return to **Jobcentre Plus**	From 24 months after attachment

Source: National Audit Office summary of the Department for Work & Pensions' Invitation to Tender (November 2010)

1.7 The Department encourages contractors to provide more support to harder-to-help groups by setting higher possible payment levels. The Department refers people to one of nine different payment groups depending on their age, benefit type and other characteristics (**Figure 3**).

1.8 Besides payments based on individual results, the Department pays incentive payments if overall performance is 30 per cent over what would have occurred without any welfare-to-work support. The incentive payment applies to three payment groups: Jobseeker's Allowance 18 to 24 (payment group 1), Jobseeker's Allowance 25 and over (payment group 2), and new Employment and Support Allowance claimants (payment group 6). The incentive payment is available for each year from 2014-15 onwards.

Figure 3
Payment groups

The Department varies payments to contractors depending on payment group

Payment group		
Number	Description	Maximum payment (excludes attachment fee)
1	Jobseeker's Allowance 18 to 24	£3,410
2	Jobseeker's Allowance 25 and over	£3,995
3	Jobseeker's Allowance early entrant	£6,200
4	Jobseeker's Allowance ex-Incapacity Benefit	£6,200
5	Employment and Support Allowance volunteer	£3,300
6	New Employment and Support Allowance claimant	£5,900
7	Employment and Support Allowance ex-Incapacity Benefit	£13,120
8	Incapacity Benefit and Income Support	£3,825
9	Jobseeker's Allowance prison leavers	£5,110

Source: Department for Work & Pensions' *Invitation to Tender,* November 2010

Competition between contractors

1.9 The Department designed the Work Programme to increase competition between contractors. It has divided England, Scotland and Wales into 18 areas, and has contracts with two or three prime contractors in each area (**Figure 4**). In total, the Department has 40 contracts for the Work Programme with 18 prime contractors which in turn have arrangements with around 700 subcontractors.

1.10 The Department has two ways to use competition to encourage performance. First it can shift levels of referrals between the contractors in an area if the difference in their performance exceeds a certain level. It has done this since August 2013. Second the Department can issue Performance Improvement Notices to prime contractors where remedial performance targets are not met and eventually terminate their contracts. The Department has a wide range of potential replacements for any contracts it terminates.

Figure 4

Contracts by geographical area

18 prime contractors manage 40 contracts over 18 areas[1]

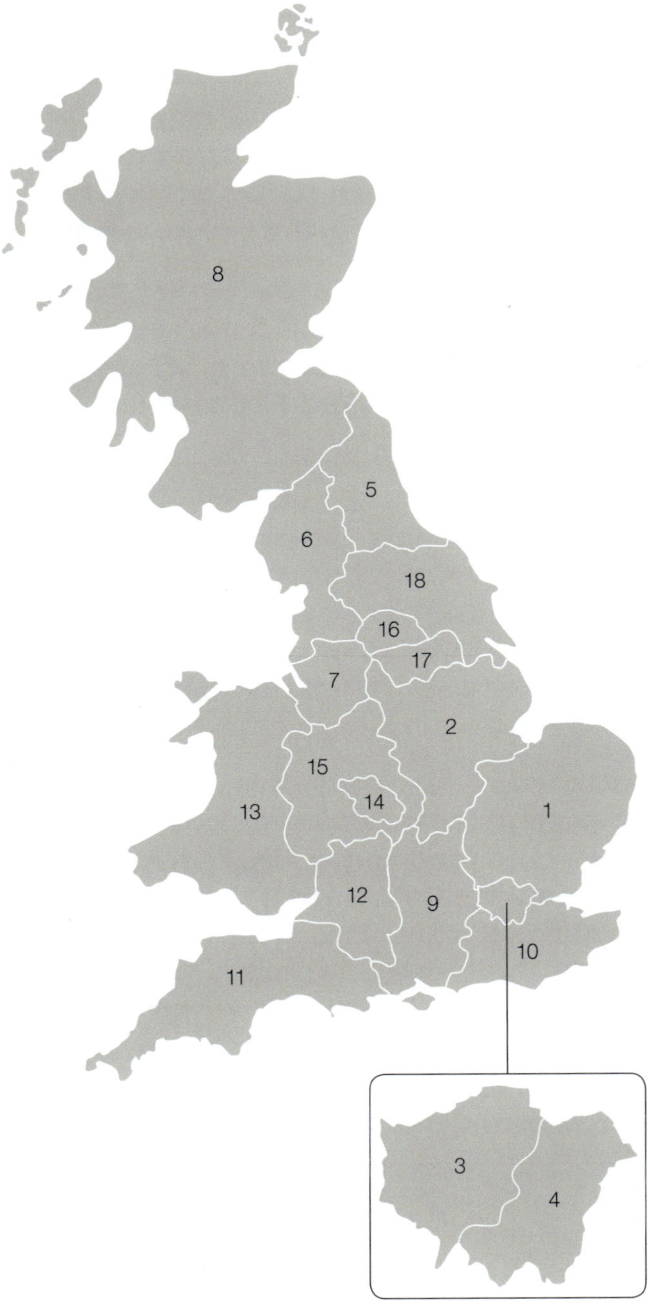

CPA 1 East of England
Ingeus
Seetec

CPA 2 East Midlands
A4e
Ingeus

CPA 3 West London
Ingeus
Maximus
Reed

CPA 4 East London
A4e
CDG
Seetec

CPA 5 North East
Avanta
Ingeus

CPA 6 North West
A4e
Ingeus

CPA 7 Greater Manchester
Avanta
G4S
Seetec

CPA 8 Scotland
Working Links
Ingeus

CPA 9 South East 1
A4e
Ingeus
Maximus

CPA 10 South East 2
Avanta
G4S

CPA 11 South West 1
Prospects
Working Links

CPA 12 South West 2
Rehab Jobfit
Learndirect

CPA 13 Wales
Rehab Jobfit
Working Links

CPA 14 Greater Birmingham
EOS-Works
Pertemps
Newcastle College Group

CPA 15 West Midlands
ESG
Serco

CPA 16 West Yorkshire
Ingeus
Interserve

CPA 17 South Yorkshire
A4e
Serco

CPA 18 North Yorkshire
G4S
Newcastle College

Notes

1. Each geographical area is known as a Contract Package Area (CPA).
2. Since June 2011, there has been a number of takeovers and mergers. For example, Interserve Working Futures took over Best, Learn Direct took over JHP, and CDG and the Shaw Trust merged.
3. In March 2014, the Department issued a notice of termination to the Newcastle College Group for its contract in Contract Package Area 18 under the voluntary break clause. The contract terminates in March 2015.

Source: National Audit Office summary of Department for Work & Pensions' contracts

A developing programme

1.11 In our January 2012 report we showed that the Department had introduced the Work Programme quickly after announcing the policy in mid-2010. The Department referred the first people to the programme in June 2011. It will make its final referrals under current contracts in March 2016 and payments could continue until March 2020 as contractors work with later participants and track outcomes.

1.12 The Department has changed the Work Programme since it was introduced. It has also made discretionary decisions, for example about Performance Improvement Notices and issuing a notice to terminate a contract (**Figure 5**). Appendix Four compares the development of the Work Programme with other major programmes we have reviewed.

1.13 Between June 2011 and March 2016 the Department expects to refer 2.1 million people to the Work Programme. By March 2014 it had referred 1.6 million people, 76 per cent of the total (**Figure 6** on page 20). Around 296,000 people had achieved job outcomes, and 687,000 had completed two years on the Work Programme.

1.14 The nature of the Work Programme is shifting, increasing the proportion of people coming from harder-to-help payment groups. At first most referrals to the Work Programme were Jobseeker's Allowance claimants. Between 2014 and 2016 the number of Jobseeker's Allowance referrals will decline, and Employment and Support Allowance claimants will account for over 40 per cent of referrals. In the rest of this report we look separately at the performance of the Work Programme for easier-to-help groups such as Jobseeker's Allowance claimants, and harder-to-help groups such as Employment and Support Allowance claimants.

1.15 We recognise that payment groups do not match directly to how hard people are to help, particularly for smaller payment groups such as Employment and Support Allowance volunteers. For the purposes of this report we refer primarily to Jobseeker's Allowance 18 to 24 (payment group 1) and Jobseeker's Allowance 25 and over (payment group 2) as examples of easier-to-help groups, and new Employment and Support Allowance claimants (payment group 6) as harder-to-help. All groups will have people who are relatively easier or harder to help and some barriers to employment (such as substance abuse) will cut across payment groups and benefit types. We have used the easier and harder-to-help distinction to help assess the Department's own aim to close gaps in performance between groups, and to reflect the changing nature of the Work Programme over time.

Figure 5
Major milestones and developments

The Work Programme has passed several milestones since June 2011

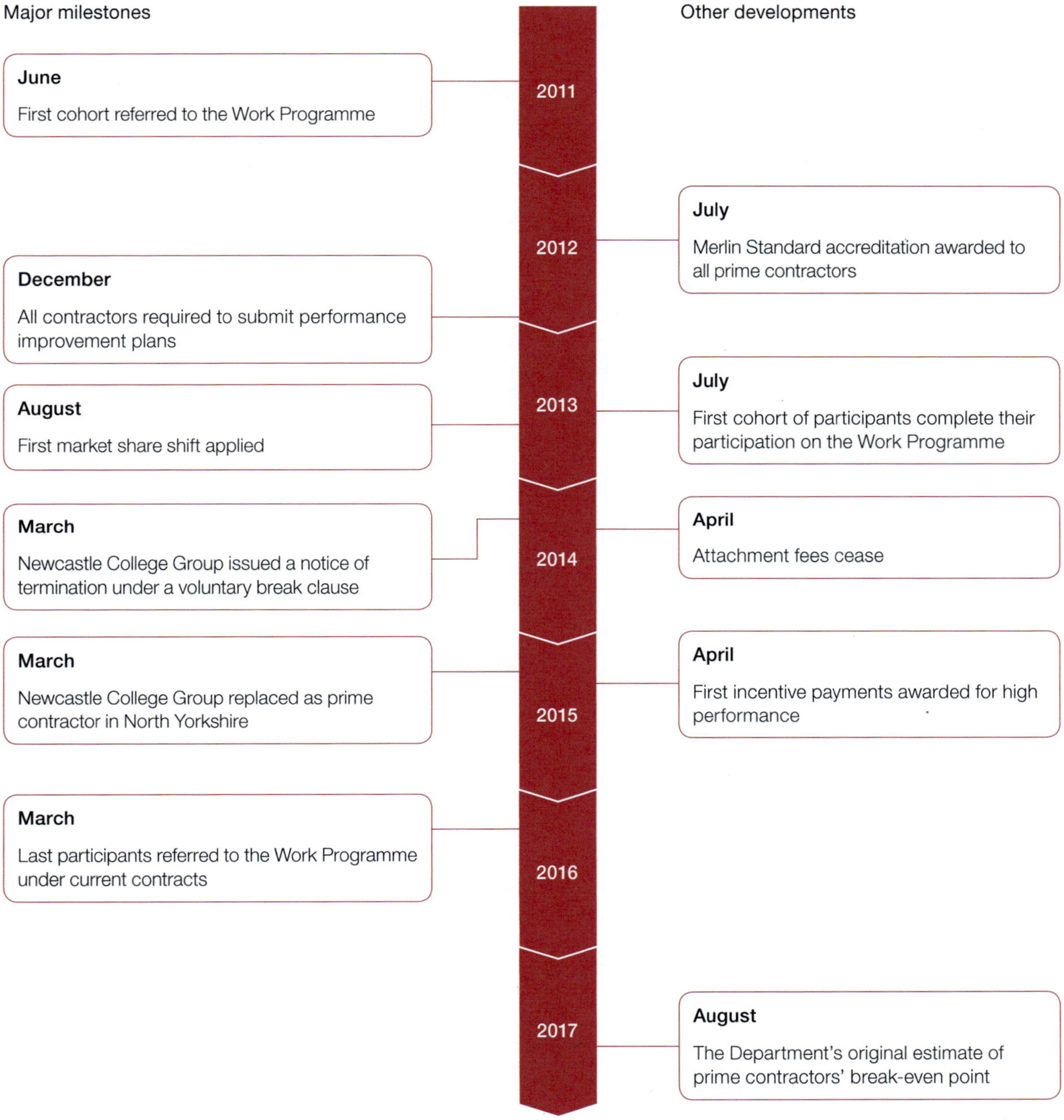

Source: National Audit Office summary of Department for Work & Pensions' documents

Figure 6
Referrals and spending

By March 2014, three-quarters of the Department's expected number of participants had been referred to the Work Programme

	Plan[1]	June 2011 to March 2014 (actual)	April 2014 to March 2020 (forecast)[2]	Total
Referrals (million)	2.4	1.6	0.5[2]	2.1
Actual or forecast spending (£ million)	3,200	1,400	1,400	2,800
Department's estimate of benefit savings compared with previous programmes (£ million)	730	20	440	450

Notes

1 The referrals for 'plan' are based on data in the Department's 'pricing model'. The values use actual prices and referral rates at expected performance levels.

2 The last referrals will be made in March 2016.

3 Some figures do not cast due to rounding.

Source: National Audit Office analysis of Department for Work & Pensions' pricing model for the Work Programme and official statistics on the Work Programme's performance

Part Two

Performance of easier-to-help groups

2.1 In this part we examine the performance of Jobseeker's Allowance claimants in the Work Programme. We look at whether the Department has:

- improved employment outcomes compared to previous programmes and the Department's expectations;
- saved money by reducing people's reliance on benefits; and
- identified ways to improve performance over time.

2.2 In most cases we use the largest payment group (Jobseeker's Allowance claimants aged 25 and over) to illustrate performance. The Department publishes a more detailed set of performance measures for each group.

Performance similar to past programmes but below expectations

2.3 The Department referred 1.3 million Jobseeker's Allowance claimants to the Work Programme up to March 2014. **Figure 7** overleaf shows the actual and forecast progress for people referred to the largest of the payment groups (Jobseeker's Allowance claimants aged 25 and over). Around 21 per cent of people had achieved job outcomes overall. Among the 316,000 people who had completed two years participation on the Work Programme this was 27 per cent.

2.4 We use the Department's information on performance to assess how the Work Programme compares to previous welfare-to-work programmes and the Department's own expectations. Outcome measures provide a broad assessment of performance. However we recognise that this is limited by: variation between payment groups; inexact comparisons with past schemes; a disproportionate impact of early cohorts of participants on performance; and uncertainty about the underlying economic environment. In Appendix Three we discuss the impact of these differences.

Figure 7

Performance for Jobseeker's Allowance claimants aged 25 and over

More recent cohorts are forecast to achieve higher performance levels

	Completed cohorts	Current and forecast cohorts[1]	Total
Referral	316,000	541,000	857,000
Attachment and support	310,000 (98 per cent)	533,000 (98 per cent)	843,000 (98 per cent)
Off benefit	40 per cent (proportion of time)	51 per cent (proportion of time)	47 per cent (proportion of time)
Job outcome achieved	85,000 (27 per cent)	205,000 (38 per cent)	290,000 (34 per cent)
Sustainment achieved	1,320,000	1,985,000	3,305,000
Completed programme without an outcome	231,000 (73 per cent)	336,000 forecast (62 per cent)	567,000 (66 per cent)

Note

1 Includes actual results to March 2014 and forecasts from April 2014 onwards.

Source: National Audit Office analysis of Department for Work & Pensions' provider payment model and its estimate of referrals; prime contractors' bids

Achieving job outcomes

2.5 The Work Programme is achieving similar levels of job outcomes to previous welfare-to-work programmes for Jobseeker's Allowance claimants aged 25 and over. Those who have completed two years participation on the Work Programme achieved a job outcome in 27 per cent of cases (**Figure 8**).

Figure 8

Performance for Jobseeker's Allowance claimants aged 25 and over – compared with expectations and previous programmes

Performance is below expectations, but similar to previous programmes

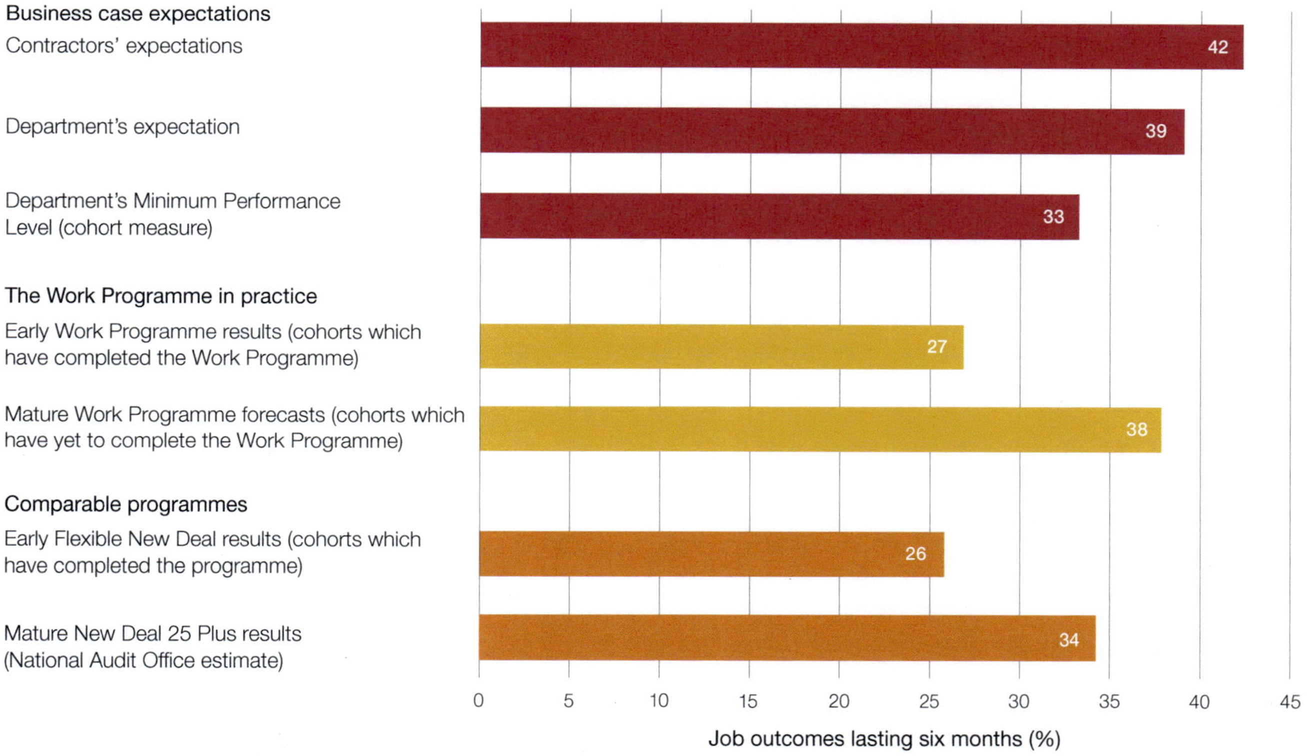

Notes

1 Contractors' expectations – estimates prime contractors submitted with bids.

2 Department's expectation – 'core' expectation used to design the Work Programme; it is not a target.

3 Department's Minimum Performance Level – expectation for each cohort's performance; contractual minimum performance levels are based on an annual snapshot so will differ.

4 Early Work Programme results – performance for cohorts that have completed two years participation on the Work Programme.

5 Mature Work Programme forecasts – expectation for cohorts not completed by April 2014.

6 Early Flexible New Deal results – Flexible New Deal performance adjusted for length and the design of the Work Programme. Three cohorts completed.

7 Mature New Deal 25 Plus results – on New Deal 25 Plus 46 per cent of individuals referred obtained a job start. The Department's analysis suggests that 80 per cent of participants kept a job for six months or more, implying a 37 per cent job outcome rate. We adjusted this further for differences in validation regimes.

Source: National Audit Office analysis of Department for Work & Pensions' provider payment model and its estimate of referrals; prime contractors' expectations of performance set out in their bids

2.6 As we described in our January 2012 report, the Department expected the Work Programme's performance to be substantially better than previous programmes.[3] The Department developed a range of estimates for performance, including a minimum performance level for Jobseeker's Allowance claimants aged 25 and over of 33 per cent over the whole course of the programme.

2.7 Early cohorts on the Work Programme have achieved similar performance to comparable cohorts on Flexible New Deal, which was a short-lived programme. The Department expects performance for Jobseeker's Allowance claimants aged 25 and over to increase to 38 per cent for remaining cohorts, achieving overall performance over the life of the Work Programme of 34 per cent.

2.8 There is variation in performance between Jobseeker's Allowance groups. People aged between 18 and 24 years perform better than older claimants. Performance for cohorts who have completed two years on the programme is 32 per cent. The Department expects this to reach 38 per cent over the Work Programme's life compared with a minimum performance level of 44 per cent.

2.9 The Department expects performance to improve in later cohorts of referrals. As we noted in our report in December 2012 the early performance of the Work Programme was well below expectations.[4] The Department's published statistics show improvement particularly for outcomes for cohorts referred in early 2012 (**Figure 9**). The Department expects this trend to continue. However, success depends heavily on how people referred since 2012 perform during their second year.

Sustaining jobs

2.10 The Work Programme seems to be as effective as previous programmes in keeping people in work for a sustained period. Between June 2011 and March 2014, the Department paid contractors around one million sustainment payments for people remaining in work beyond six months. Using the Department's assumptions we compared the rate of sustainment payments for Jobseeker's Allowance claimants over 25 years old with the performance of those on New Deal 25 Plus and found similar levels of performance in sustaining jobs beyond the first six months (**Figure 10** on page 26).

2.11 Jobseeker's Allowance claimants aged 18 to 24 sustain work better than comparable participants in New Deal. Between June 2011 and March 2014, the Department paid contractors around 500,000 sustainment payments for people still in work beyond six months for this group. The Work Programme has achieved 27 per cent more sustained months of employment compared to the New Deal.

3 Comptroller and Auditor General, *The introduction of the Work Programme*, Session 2011-12, HC 1701, National Audit Office, January 2012.

4 Comptroller and Auditor General, *A commentary for the Committee of Public Accounts on the Work Programme outcome statistics*, Session 2012-13, HC 832, National Audit Office, December 2012.

Figure 9
Jobseeker's Allowance claimants aged 25 and over – cohort performance over time

Performance improved for cohorts starting in early 2012 and early 2013

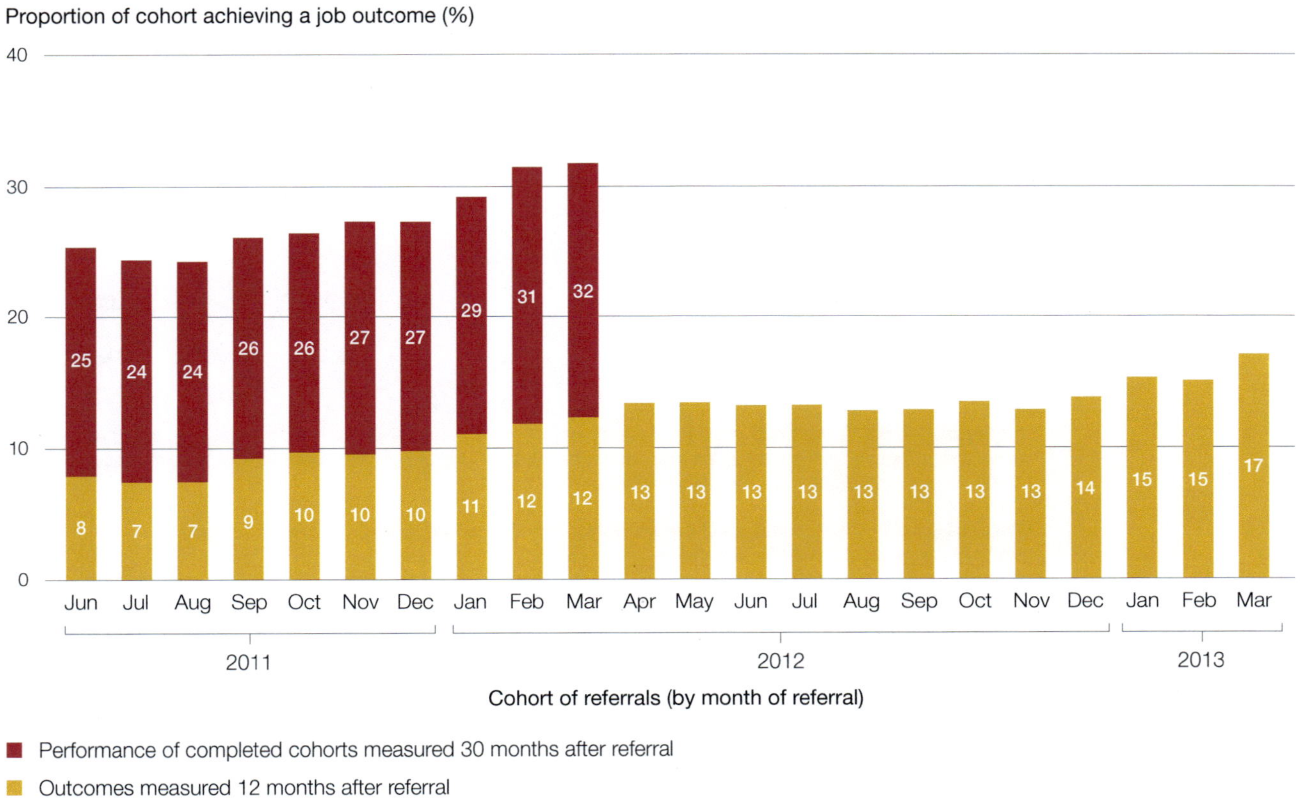

Note

1 Performance of completed cohorts – cohorts for November 2011 to March 2012 have completed two years participation, but performance is measured 30 months after referral to include participants starting employment in the final months. We have included small and stable estimates for these participants for the last five cohorts.

Source: National Audit Office analysis of the Department for Work & Pensions' published performance data

Figure 10

Sustaining employment – Jobseeker's Allowance claimants aged 25 and over

Participants sustained employment at a similar level to the Department's estimate of previous programmes

	June 2011 to March 2014	Forecast for the Work Programme
National Audit Office estimate of valid sustainment payments	1,015,000	3,121,000
Equivalent estimate of sustainment payments on previous programmes[1]	989,000	3,041,000
Difference	**26,000**	**80,000**
	3%	**3%**

Note

1 National Audit Office estimate using the Department for Work & Pensions' analysis of previous programmes and adjusting for a modelling error which informed the Invitation to Tender. The error understated sustainment payments 20 per cent by volume and £300 million by value.

Source: National Audit Office analysis of Department for Work & Pensions' provider payment model and its pricing model; and published official statistics

Under-reported outcomes

2.12 Measured performance is based on job outcomes claimed by contractors and validated by the Department. Several contractors told us that they had not been able to claim job outcomes for people they suspected but could not demonstrate were in work. In this case measured performance would understate the actual success of the Work Programme.

2.13 The Department has estimated how many job outcomes are hidden in this way. It identified people who had long spells off benefit but for whom no job outcome had been claimed. It then used real time information on earnings from HM Revenue & Customs to estimate how many of these people were actually in work. The Department estimates that around 26,000 people satisfied conditions for job outcomes between June 2011 and December 2013 but for whom contractors had not made a job outcome claim, around 9 per cent of the total number of job outcomes claimed up to the end of 2013.

2.14 The Department is not able to break down its estimate into specific cohorts and performance over time. We have not validated the methodology. It is not clear whether unreported outcomes arise because contractors are unaware of outcomes or avoid making claims that might fail and be penalised in the validation process.

Less time on benefit

2.15 People are spending less time on benefit than the Department expected given the number of job outcomes achieved. For Jobseeker's Allowance claimants over 25 years old the Department has reduced its initial forecast for job outcomes by 15 per cent. But based on experience so far it has only reduced its forecast for people coming off benefit by 9 per cent. It is not clear whether the initial expectation for time off benefit was pessimistic, or whether more people are coming off benefit without work.

2.16 The disparity between time off benefit and outcomes is even higher in other payment groups. Across all payment groups the Department estimates the Work Programme will reduce benefit spending by £450 million against the baseline agreed with HM Treasury.

Improving performance

2.17 Contractors have also highlighted positive aspects of the Work Programme and the potential for improving performance further. Contractors told us that they benefited from more available information about outcomes, from engaging with the Department's staff and opportunities for sharing good practice (**Figure 11** overleaf).

2.18 Claimants and other stakeholders have raised a number of concerns about the quality of support provided in the Work Programme. These include: referring people to inappropriate training and using sanctions as a way to push people into finding work; pressuring people to take jobs that they are not suited for; discriminating inappropriately between people in the way support is allocated; and failing to take account of an individual's needs and circumstances.

2.19 The Department has commissioned a consortium of third party experts to undertake a multi-year evaluation of the Work Programme and assess the kinds of issues raised by claimants and contractors. The Department published early evaluation reports looking at programme delivery and commissioning, in November 2012 and March 2013. The Department has postponed the release of some interim evaluation findings based on claimant and contractor surveys. It now plans to publish a more extensive set of evaluation findings in late 2014.

Figure 11

Prime contractors' views – easier-to-help groups

Prime contractors have identified positive aspects of the Work Programme and areas for improvement

	Examples of what is working well	Examples of areas for improvement
Referral	Jobcentre Plus offices co-located with contractors to ensure 'warm handovers'	Inaccurate forecasts from the Department hinder contractors' ability to plan and invest The Department did not apply the market shift mechanism to two areas because participants had not been treated equally
Attachment and support	Quarterly Provider Forum for contractors to share ideas and best practice	Compliance methodology limits the Department's ability to identify 'parking' Compliance data is not analysed thematically, nor shared with providers in order to add value
Off benefit	Provider Direct telephone helpline updates contractors about participants' circumstances Department's off-benefit reports help contractors validate claims, and identify participants falling out of work	Inaccuracies with the Department's off-benefit check means some valid claims are rejected, although the Department believe the number is very low
Job outcome achieved	Department's Provider Assurance Teams give constructive recommendations Department has a thorough system for validating claims and allowing contractors to challenge	Department's validation team do not communicate effectively with contractors to improve claim accuracy Guidance for validating self-employed claims is unclear
Sustainment achieved	Department changed evidence requirements for validation to reduce the burden on prime contractors	Number of sustainment payments is burdensome for contractors, employers, and the Department to validate
Completed programme without an outcome		Exit reports are not provided consistently and if produced for more participants would provide a good measure of achievement while on the Work Programme

Source: National Audit Office summary of providers' responses

Part Three

Performance of harder-to-help groups

3.1 The Department intends that the Work Programme will narrow the gap in employment rates between easier and harder-to-help groups and reduce the levels of parking of the harder-to-help. In this part we look at whether the Department has:

- improved employment outcomes compared to previous programmes and the Department's expectations; and
- encouraged contractors to support harder-to-help groups effectively.

Similar performance to previous programmes

3.2 The Department referred 262,000 Employment and Support Allowance claimants to the Work Programme from June 2011 to March 2014. **Figure 12** overleaf shows the progress of people referred to the largest payment group, new Employment and Support Allowance claimants.

3.3 Overall the Work Programme has not improved performance for Employment and Support Allowance claimants. The Department set a minimum performance level for new claimants of Employment and Support Allowance of 22 per cent, which the Department now accepts was too high. Only 11 per cent of participants who have completed the Work Programme have secured a job outcome. The Department forecasts that this will rise to 14 per cent by the end of the Work Programme. Performance is below what prime contractors expected when they bid and is broadly similar to that of previous comparable welfare-to-work initiatives (**Figure 13** on page 31).

3.4 In November 2012, the Department broadened the criteria for new claimants of Employment and Support Allowance. Originally, people who the Department assessed as being ready for work within six months were referred to the Work Programme. The Department expanded referrals to those with 12 month prognoses and it expects 100,000 of these up to March 2016. The Department forecasts that 7 per cent of people with 12 month prognoses will achieve a job outcome while those with a shorter prognosis will secure job outcomes in 16 per cent of cases for cohorts yet to complete the programme.

Figure 12

Performance for new Employment and Support Allowance claimants

Eleven per cent of new Employment and Support Allowance claimants completing the Work Programme have secured a job outcome

	Completed cohorts	Current and forecast cohorts	Total
Referral	41,000	289,000	330,000
Attachment and support	40,000 (97 per cent)	281,000 (97 per cent)	321,000 (97 per cent)
Off benefit	18 per cent (proportion of time)	25 per cent (proportion of time)	24 per cent (proportion of time)
Job outcome achieved	5,000 (11 per cent)	40,000 (14 per cent)	45,000 (14 per cent)
Sustainment achieved	105,000	577,000	682,000
Completed programme without an outcome	36,000 (89 per cent)	249,000 forecast (86 per cent)	285,000 (86 per cent)

Notes

1 'Current and forecast cohorts' includes actual results to March 2014 and the Department's forecasts.

2 'Current and forecast cohorts' includes Employment and Support Allowance claimants with a 12 month prognosis who were referred from November 2012. They constitute a third of forecast referrals and are more difficult to help than participants with a three or six month prognosis.

Source: National Audit Office analysis of Department for Work & Pensions' provider payments model and its estimate of referrals

Figure 13

Performance for new Employment and Support Allowance claimants – compared with expectations and previous programmes

Performance for harder-to-help participants is currently behind expectations

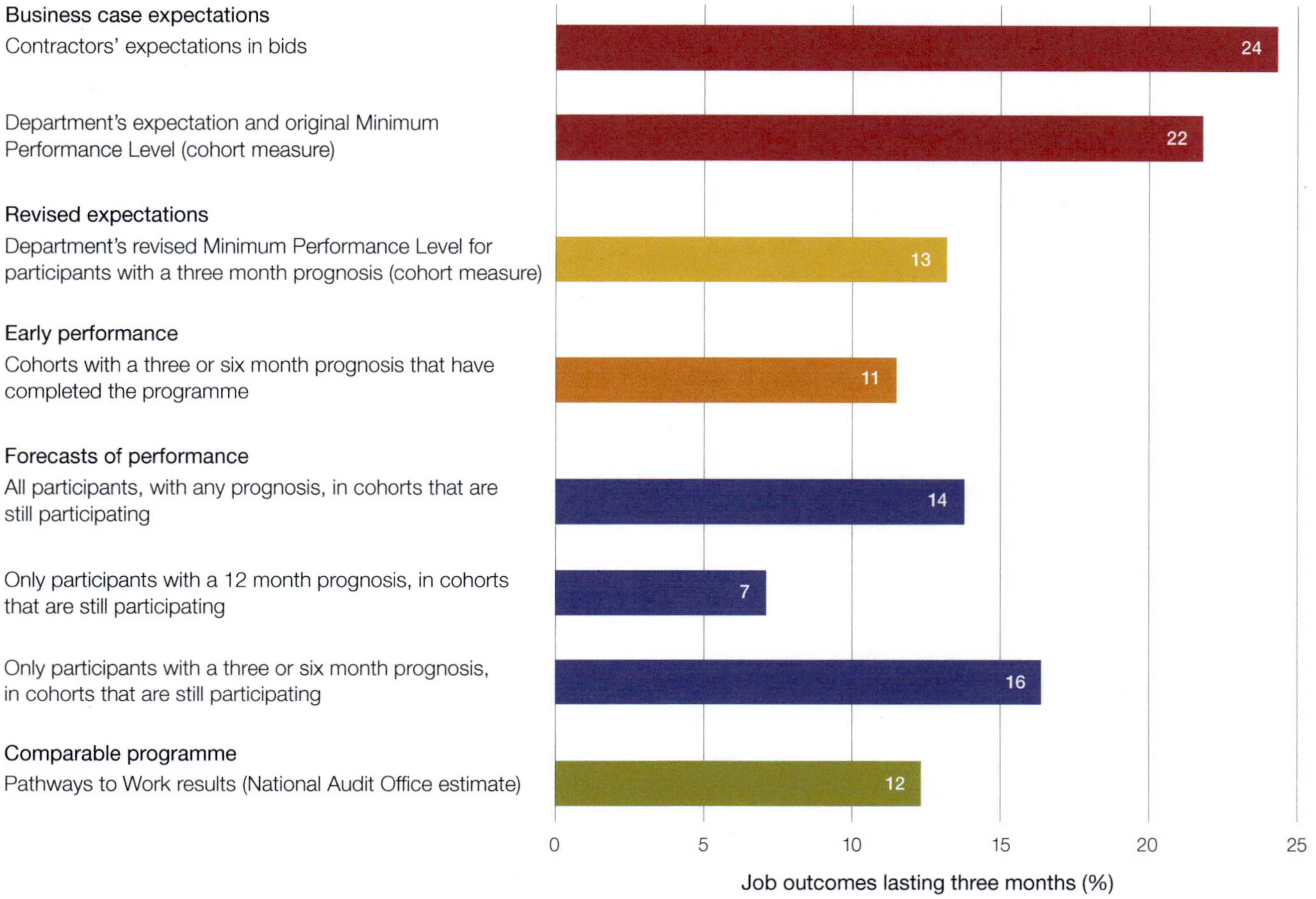

Notes

1 Contractors' expectations – expectations based on participants with a three month prognosis only; and taken from the prime contractors' bids.

2 Department's expectation and original minimum performance level – 'core' expectation based on participants with a three month prognosis only. Contractual minimum performance levels are based on an annual snapshot so will differ.

3 Department's revised Minimum Performance Level – revised estimate now that more data is available for participants with a three or six month prognosis. For participants with a 12 month prognosis it is 7 per cent.

4 Early Work Programme results – cohorts starting between June 2011 and March 2012 with a three or six month prognosis.

5 Mature Work Programme forecasts – includes Employment and Support Allowance claimants with a 12 month prognosis who were referred to Work Programme from November 2012. The Department forecasts that a third of referrals will have a 12 month prognosis.

6 Pathways to Work – includes all Incapacity Benefit claimants, so there is no distinction between prognoses. Pathways to Work measured job starts not three month job outcomes. On Pathways to Work 15 per cent of mandatory referrals to contractor-led services obtained a job start. The Department's analysis suggest that 88 per cent of participants maintain a job for three months or longer, implying a job outcome rate of 13 per cent. We adjusted this further for differences in validation regimes.

Source: National Audit Office analysis of Department for Work & Pensions' performance data

3.5 The Department's published performance data shows that the performance of later cohorts of referrals is improving (**Figure 14**). The Department expects the improvement to continue but still forecasts performance to fall short of its initial expectations.

3.6 The Department estimates that 2,000 of the 26,000 additional job outcomes it recently identified related to Employment and Support Allowance claimant groups.

Reducing spending on the harder-to-help group

3.7 The Department was concerned by 'parking' harder-to-help participants on previous welfare-to-work schemes. In designing the Work Programme it set higher payments for job outcomes in harder-to-help groups. The Department's intention was to encourage prime contractors to increase their targeting of and spending on support for participants with higher barriers to employment.

3.8 The spending prime contractors allocate to harder-to-help payment groups has reduced by on average 54 per cent per person from their original bids. We reviewed estimates from 20 contracts. Compared to an average of £1,360 when they bid, these contractors now expect to spend £630 per person on new Employment and Support Allowance claimants. This amount is lower than their expected spending per person – £870 – for the largest Jobseeker's Allowance payment group.

3.9 We identified three factors which influence how much prime contractors spend on harder-to-help groups.

- **Less targeting by payment group.** Payment groups have not encouraged all contractors to target services at harder-to-help participants in the way intended. Some contractors have always allocated spending based on a participant's payment group; others have recently adopted a targeted approach in response to the increasing proportion of referrals of Employment and Support Allowance claimants. Other contractors allocate services to suit the needs of the individual which they believe is not captured by payment groups.

- **Expected funding has reduced.** Prime contractors argue that average funding for participants claiming Employment and Support Allowance is less than those on Jobseeker's Allowance when actual performance levels are considered.

- **Changes to services.** Prime contractors told us they have adapted services since they made their bids, some of which require less spending. For example, the introduction of participants that are further from employment has allowed greater use of group work or 'lighter touch', less frequent contact which can be more appropriate to their needs.

Figure 14
New Employment and Support Allowance claimants (3 or 6 month prognoses) – cohort performance over time

Performance for later cohorts has improved

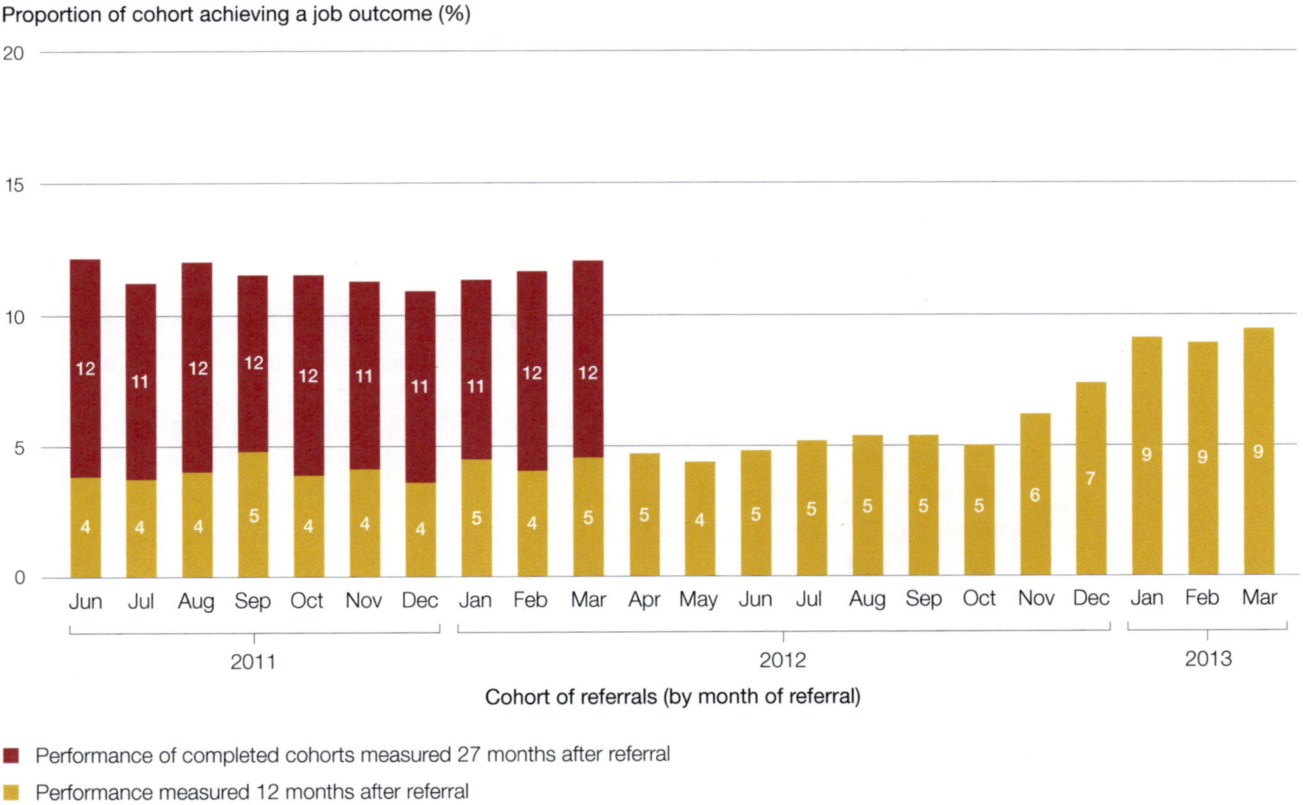

Notes

1 Excludes 12 month prognosis claimants.

2 Performance of completed cohorts – cohorts for November 2011 to March 2012 have completed two years participation, but performance is measured 27 months after referral to include participants starting employment in the final months. We have included small and stable estimates for these participants for the last two cohorts (February and March 2012).

Source: National Audit Office analysis of Department for Work & Pensions' published performance data

Limited monitoring of levels of support

3.10 The Department has not set out the levels of support it considers each contractor should give people. Instead the Department asked prime contractors to set their own minimum service standards in their bids to help guarantee service quality regulators of employment barriers. In total, the 18 contractors set 212 minimum service standards. Only four of the 18 contractors set minimum service standards that differentiate between different groups of participants.

3.11 In the absence of useable minimum performance standards, data on caseloads provides an indicator of changes in services. Between December 2011 and June 2013, the average number of participants a case worker supported increased steadily from 122 to 154. By December 2013, it dropped back to 117 as fewer people are now on the programme.

3.12 In response to the difficulty of monitoring and enforcing minimum service standards the Department has changed how it oversees contractor performance (**Figure 15**).

3.13 The Department's Compliance Monitoring Officers have been in place since the start of the Work Programme. They use the contractors' minimum services standards and a set of 14 standardised quality measures to monitor each prime contractor's service quality. Each month, the Compliance Monitoring Officers randomly test 1,000 individual case files.

3.14 The Department's approach could be helpful to identify 'parking'. The latest analysis shows that 46 per cent of participants had not had contact with their contractor in the last two months. However, the data is poorly defined and is not an effective test of parking. The 1,000 case files are taken from all participants since the start of the Work Programme in June 2011. The sample therefore does not account for those people who have left the Work Programme and would therefore not be in contact with the prime contractor. The Department does not consider the participant's payment group as part of its analysis.

Figure 15
Minimum service standards and monitoring timeline

The Department has changed its approach to monitoring services

	Development
June 2011	Monitoring and managing performance against bid commitments: • Contractors agree minimum service standards with the Department based on their bids • Department set 14 generic key control questions • Compliance Monitoring Officers introduced
June 2013	A single point of guidance for step-by-step processes: • New Performance Management Regime introduced setting out the structure and level of interventions the Department will have with contractors, including the introduction of Performance Improvement Notices for poorer performing contractors
July 2013	A quantitative approach to monitoring: • New approach to compliance scoring
August 2013	Rewarding better performing contractors and encouraging others to improve: • Market share shift introduced
January 2014	A regional structure for managing performance: • Revised Work Programme Performance Management regime
April 2014	Checking end-to-end process: • Assurance Officer role introduced

Source: National Audit Office analysis of Department for Work & Pensions' performance management information and interviews with officials

Improving performance

3.15 For harder to help groups, contractors have highlighted aspects of the Work Programme that work well and those the Department might improve (**Figure 16**).

Figure 16

Prime Contractors' views – harder-to-help groups

Contractors have identified positive aspects of the Work Programme and areas for improvement

Stage	Examples of what is working well	Examples of areas for improvement
Referral	Support from the Provider Direct telephone helpline helps to track participants who have not engaged	Introduction of 12-month prognosis Employment and Support Allowance claimants in 2012 affected prime contractors' investment decisions Increasing proportion of Employment and Support Allowance claimants when attachment fees are decreasing puts strain on contractors' working capital
Attachment and support	Increased length of time participants spend on the Work Programme gives contractors more time to tackle barriers for the hardest to help	The Department can take up to 12 months to agree changes to minimum service levels
Off benefit		
Job outcome achieved	Recognising cumulative rather than continuous employment has improved participants' ability to get an outcome	The introduction of Employment and Support Allowance 12 month prognosis participants has not been reflected in the minimum performance level requirements, yet they are a group with many more challenges to address
Sustainment achieved		Given the complex barriers some participants face, one provider suggested it would be helpful to move some funding from sustainment payments to the attachment stage for these groups in order for contractors to invest in the full suite of services needed to move these participants into work
Completed programme without an outcome		Exit reports are not provided consistently. All participants returned to Jobcentre Plus require an exit report. However, those who sign off benefit or find work do not. An exit report for all participants would be a good measure of progression

Source: National Audit Office summary of providers' response to consultation

Part Four

Controlling costs

4.1 To control costs effectively, the Department needs to show: it is paying a reasonable amount for the services contractors provide; it does not pay for unconfirmed services or outcomes; and that it measures and rewards contractors in a way that encourages performance. In this part we look at how the Department has affected costs by the way it:

- transfers performance risks to contractors;
- validates outcomes before making payments; and
- manages overall contractor performance.

Lower financial risk for government

4.2 The Department's payment-by-results approach has reduced some of the risks to government of low performance. The Department expected to pay contractors £1.7 billion between June 2011 and March 2014. It actually paid contractors £1.4 billion (83 per cent) because there were fewer outcomes than expected (**Figure 17** overleaf). The Committee of Public Accounts has previously highlighted that while this reduces the risk to government from poor performance it does not pass risks fully to contractors.

4.3 Partly because of risk sharing the Department has spent less on the Work Programme than it would have done on previous programmes. It is difficult to make direct comparisons with past programmes. Based on its own modelling the Department expects to spend £41 million less on the Work Programme between June 2011 and March 2020 than it would have done for similar levels of performance on previous welfare-to-work programmes.

Figure 17
Transferring risk to contractors

Outcome based payments reduce the cost to the Department of poor performance

	Department's expectation (June 2011 to March 2014)	Actual (June 2011 to March 2014)	Change (%)
Outcomes achieved	418,000	296,000	-29
Attachment payments (£m)	538	538	0
Job outcome payments (£m)	464	334	-28
Sustainment payments (£m)	700	503	-28
Total payments (£m)	**1,702**	**1,375**	**-19**
Cost per outcome	**£4,074**	**£4,650**	**14**

Source: Analysis of Department for Work & Pensions' Provider Payment model and its performance information

Lower profits for contractors

4.4 Contractors now expect to make much lower profits than in their original bids for the Work Programme. In 2013, prime contractors responsible for 35 of the 40 contracts submitted forecasts of revenue and costs for the Work Programme's life to the Department. Total profits were 57 per cent lower than they originally expected. Revenue and profits are lower as a result of lower performance and lower than anticipated referrals. Prime contractors told us that they considered the Work Programme was currently viable, but that they had concerns about the future. They also questioned the viability of the Work Programme as a stand-alone contract.

4.5 The Department has not changed payment terms to relieve the pressure on contractors as it did for Flexible New Deal contracts. The original payment terms remain, including discounts on job outcome payments that contractors offered in their bids. In our January 2012 report *Introduction of the Work Programme*, we identified a risk that contractors might face problems of financial sustainability. There is little evidence that this has affected contractors so far.

4.6 One possible response to low performance is that contractors might try to reduce costs, particularly by reducing subcontracted services, changing terms, or closing support centres. Contractors estimate that overall costs have reduced by 12 per cent in response to lower volumes. But spending on subcontractors has fallen by 24 per cent. The Department has not completed any analysis to assess the impact of the reduction in funding in these areas.

4.7 The main reason for reduced spending on subcontractors appears to be fewer than expected harder-to-help referrals in early stages of the Work Programme. Up to March 2014, 262,000 people claiming Employment and Support Allowance were referred to prime contractors – 55 per cent of the level contractors assumed in their bids.

4.8 No contractor has breached the Department's standards for supply chain management. The Department independently accredits prime contractors against the Merlin Standard, the Department's code of conduct for relationships between subcontractors and prime contractors. Contractors are given a rating of 'excellent', 'good', 'satisfactory', or 'unacceptable'. There are 12 contracts held by contractors with a 'satisfactory' rating, and 28 with a 'good' rating. Although individual subcontractors left the programme there is no indication of market failure. The Department's evaluation found the prime contractors' supply chains had a 10 per cent 'churn' annually.

Need to improve validation

4.9 The Department validates contractors' claims for job outcome payments and sustainment payments. It uses a series of checks including comparing claims to records of taxes and benefits, and testing samples of specific claims in detail (**Figure 18** overleaf).

Improved validation of job outcome payments

4.10 The Department has set up an extensive set of checks on job outcomes, which the Committee of Public Accounts has recognised as improving on previous contracted programmes.[5] The Department has established a dedicated team, the Provider Payment Validation Team, to check a sample of contractors' claims. In 2013-14 it failed 7 per cent of the job outcome claims it reviewed. Up to March 2014 the Department has saved £21 million by extrapolating invalid job outcome payments and reducing payments to contractors accordingly.

5 HC Committee of Public Accounts, *Preventing fraud in contracted employment programmes*, Fifteenth Report of Session 2012-13, HC 103.

Figure 18

Job outcome and sustainment payment validation

The Department uses two different approaches to validating claims

Description of claim	Job outcome payments	Sustainment payments
Timing	After 13 or 26 weeks of employment depending on payment group	For additional 28 days of employment after job outcome
Claims per participant	Up to 1 per participant	Up to 13 to 26 per participant depending on the payment group
Total claims	Total expected: 0.6 million Up to March 2014: 0.3 million	Total expected: 7.2 million Up to March 2014: 2.4 million
Value of claims	Total expected: £0.7 billion Up to March 2014: £0.3 billion	Total expected: £1.6 billion Up to March 2014: £0.5 billion
Validation step		
Off-benefit check	100 per cent of claims checked pre-payment Around 5 per cent fail	100 per cent of claims checked pre-payment Around 5 per cent fail
HMRC check	100 per cent of off-benefit claims checked Around 35 per cent pass	Not checked; data not available monthly
Payment validation sample	Sample taken by payment validation team Estimate valid claims for each contractor Claims assessed as pass, fail, technical fail or unable to validate	Sample taken by payment validation team Estimate valid claims overall Claims assessed as pass, fail, technical fail or unable to validate
Challenge and resubmit	Contractor can challenge assessment on individual sampled claims Contractor can resubmit claim at a future date if failed	No challenge process given lack of claw back and extrapolation Contractor can resubmit claim at any time if it has failed
Claw back	Payments reduced by contractor's sampled fail rate (after challenge) extrapolated across all contractor's claims	Payments reduced only by the specific claims that fail in sample; no extrapolation

Note

1 Off-benefit check involves comparing claims with records of benefit payments in the Department's CIS database.

Source: National Audit Office review of Department for Work & Pensions' data and documents

4.11 The Department is continuing to improve its approach to validating job outcomes. It has removed requirements to get permission before contacting employers and has learnt how to elicit more accurate information about employment. One particularly difficult issue is how to treat claims the Department is 'unable to validate', for example if employers do not respond to enquiries. At the moment the Department treats these claims as valid claims. By improving validation the Department has reduced the share of claims it is unable to validate and it is considering how to apportion claims between valid and invalid claims in future.

4.12 An external review of the validation process gives some assurance about the accuracy of the Department's estimates of invalid claims. The Department commissioned PricewaterhouseCoopers (PwC) to test a sample of claims and compare results with the Department's own estimates. Although PwC failed a higher proportion of claims in the sample, it is likely that the difference is largely due to differences in methodology. Where a contractor's information about a claim is wrong the Department's team goes to greater lengths to establish whether a job outcome has actually occurred.

Sustainment payments losses

4.13 Sustainment payments are more difficult for the Department to validate. It is harder to design a statistically valid sample of claims when there could be several claims per participant. Contractors also find that employers become increasingly frustrated by having to confirm employees' details up to a maximum of 27 times, leading to poor quality information about participants.

4.14 The Department did not include an extrapolated 'claw back' of invalid sustainment payments in Work Programme contracts. Unlike for job outcome claims, the Department cannot reduce sustainment payments in proportion to the invalid claims it samples. The Department has not had a clear and consistent approach to validating sustainment payments. It is not clear why the Department did not include the option to extrapolate invalid claims in the original contracts. The Department has also relaxed requirements for contractors to confirm that participants are in employment.

4.15 The Department estimates that around 7 per cent of sustainment payment claims fail validation, but does not have a statistically valid estimate for each contractor individually. Claims that fail the validation process may relate to people who are in work but whose details are not up to date. Using real time information data from HM Revenue & Customs, the Department estimates over 75 per cent of failed claims do relate to valid sustainment outcomes. This is consistent with the views of contractors who have done their own re-checking of valid claims.

4.16 Based on its estimates of valid claims and the more recent real time information data the Department estimates that it paid £11 million up to March 2014 for sustainment payments that it is unlikely to be able to validate. These payments are defined as losses, because the Department has paid for services or outcomes it has not received.

4.17 As we approach the later stages of the Work Programme sustainment payments are becoming an increasingly large share of total payments. The Department expects that they will cost £1 billion over the rest of the Work Programme. Assuming no change to the validation regime and a similar level of invalid payments the future cost would be around £25 million.

4.18 The Department has recognised the importance of improving the validation of sustainment payments. Over the past year it has examined the validation regime, including asking PwC to test a sample of claims in response to Cabinet Office concerns about payment validation. The Department has developed a new method for estimating invalid payments for each contractor. It is also discussing future changes to the validation regime with contractors. It is possible that the Department will need to offset the impact of extrapolating invalid sustainment payments by increasing other payments to contractors.

Flawed basis for measuring contractual performance

4.19 The Department's primary measure for contract management is the minimum performance level measure. This is the ratio between job outcomes and referrals, and *over the whole course* of the Work Programme will give a summary measure of each contractor's performance. Work Programme contracts specify the minimum performance levels contractors must achieve in the three largest payment groups.

4.20 Unfortunately the minimum performance level measure is not a good measure to use *during the programme*. By comparing current outcomes with current referrals the measure is highly sensitive to changes in referral volumes over time. As referral volumes have declined this has led to an increase in the measure across all contractors that is unrelated to underlying performance.

Over-rewarding contractors

4.21 The flaws in the minimum performance level measure mean that the Department will have to make substantial incentive payments to contractors. Incentive payments are supposed to reward very high performance by prime contractors. But in 2014-15 the Department expects that all 40 contracts will meet the level needed to trigger incentive payments because lower than expected referrals have inflated the performance measure. In 2014-15, the Department estimated that it could pay contractors £31 million, with its total potential exposure up to 2017-18 of almost £61 million. If the Department had a more accurate measure of performance, payments would be £6 million in 2014-15 and £17 million in total.

Difficulty performance managing contractors

4.22 The minimum performance level measure makes it difficult to differentiate between contractors and manage performance. The Department can shift market share between contractors if one contractor performs much better than another in an area. But the original Work Programme contracts only allowed market share shift if the better contractor was achieving minimum performance levels. In the early stages of the Work Programme all contractors struggled to meet minimum performance levels. The Department had to introduce changes to contracts to remove this restriction on market share shift.

Costly termination of contracts

4.23 In March 2014, the Department announced that it would terminate the contract with the Newcastle College Group in North Yorkshire. Newcastle College Group is required to operate within the terms of the contract for the next twelve months while the Department appoints a replacement prime contractor. The Department decided this based on a range of measures including relative contractor performance and costs.

4.24 The Department assessed Newcastle College Group as under-performing. However, it could not argue that the prime contractor had breached its contract and failed to meet minimum performance levels. Instead the Department issued its notice of termination under the voluntary break clause in the contract. It is too early to say whether the termination of the contract with the Newcastle College Group will lead to improved contractor performance.

Many changes to contracts and performance management

4.25 Since 2011 the Department has taken an active approach to changing contracts and how it manages contractor performance. The Department recognises that the rolling out the Work Programme quickly has meant that it has had to make changes while the Work Programme is running. In the period June 2011 to March 2014, the Department made 30 changes to its contract (**Figure 19** overleaf).

4.26 The Department is unlikely to be able to recover all of the costs resulting from the flaws in the design of performance measures or sustainment payments. But it has estimated that its actions since June 2011 could save £40 million over the Work Programme's life. Changes may also lead to better support and outcomes for participants.

4.27 The Department has used discretionary action when contracts have not allowed it to manage performance effectively. The Department, after realising that the formal performance management measures were ineffective, set up a bespoke process to assess whether to terminate poorly performing contracts. It expects that the termination will encourage other contractors to improve performance.

Figure 19
Variations to contracts – June 2011 to March 2014

The Department has achieved potential costs savings of £40 million by varying the terms and conditions of its contracts

Changes to improve performance	Impact
Termination of a contract with poor 'overall delivery'	Saving anticipated
Remove requirement for contracts to meet minimum performance levels in all three payment groups in order to gain referrals in the first Market Share Shift	Nine Contract Package Areas had referrals shifted between contracts from August 2013 Cost neutral
Assess the weakest 25 per cent of contractors, rather than contractors that fail to meet minimum performance levels	Undetermined by the Department
Contractors given new powers to issue sanctions to participants that do not participate in specific activities	Increase in the number of sanctions
Change to improve quality of services	**Impact**
Introduce 14 objective generic tests to assess service quality (12 of which recognised in contracts)	Undetermined by the Department
Enable performance managers to investigate specific problems reported	Undetermined by the Department
Changes to administrative burden on contractors	**Impact**
Reduce evidence requirement for sustainment payments	Reduce contractor costs Potentially increase unsupported claims for sustainment payments
Changes to improve validation of outcome claims	**Impact**
Remove the requirement for a contractor to give permission to the Department to contact a participant	'Unable to validate' rates fallen 25 per cent to 11 per cent of sampled claims
Contractual changes to 2014	Cost avoidance of £40 million

Source: Summary of meetings with Department for Work & Pensions

Appendix One

Our audit approach

1 This report compares performance of the Work Programme to previous welfare-to-work programmes and the Department's aims. We considered in particular the Department's: performance for easier-to-help groups; performance for harder-to-help groups; and its success in controlling costs. Our audit approach is summarised in **Figure 20** overleaf.

2 We considered two benchmarks for value for money related to the Department's stated aims to improve on past programmes and achieve higher levels of performance. First we considered how the Work Programme compares with previous programmes in terms of performance and costs. Second we compared performance to the Department's expectations for the programme. Where the Department has not been explicit about its intentions we have made a judgment about what a reasonable outcome would have been, for example in controlling costs. **Figure 21** on page 47 maps the findings of the report against different performance and cost criteria, and the two benchmarks.

Figure 20
Our audit approach

Government objectives

The Department introduced the Work Programme to replace existing welfare-to-work programmes that it considered performed poorly. In designing the Work Programme, the Department sought to: get more people into work and keep them there; decrease average time spent on benefit; narrow the gap between disadvantaged groups and others.

How this will be achieved

The Department refers people to contractors who provide employment support over 2 years. The Department pays contractors largely based on their success in getting people into work. Payment levels differ depending on participants' payment groups. The Department also manages performance directly against minimum performance levels.

Our study examines

The performance of the Work Programme up to March 2014 in terms of getting people into work and in particular supporting harder-to-help groups, and also the success of the Department in controlling costs.

Our evaluative criteria

The Department is meeting its expectations in getting easier-to-help groups into work.

The Department is meeting its aims to improve outcomes for harder-to-help groups.

The Department is controlling costs and reducing risks to government spending.

Our evidence

We assessed performance for Jobseeker's Allowance payment groups based on:

- Departmental performance data.
- Departmental models of previous programme performance.
- Departmental estimates from business cases.
- Contractors' estimates in bids.
- Interviews with Departmental officials and contractors.

We assessed performance for Employment and Support Allowance payment groups based on:

- Departmental data and models as for easier-to-help groups.
- Departmental data and contractual references to minimum services.
- Interviews with Departmental officials and contractors.

We assessed the Department's approach to controlling costs by:

- Interviewing Departmental officials and contractors.
- Visiting five provider sites with our financial auditors to review payment controls.
- Reviewing contractors' estimates of revenues and costs.

Our conclusion

Performance – which is improving and may be understated – is similar to previous programmes but below the levels the Department originally expected. The Work Programme has not improved performance for harder-to-help groups or closed the gap with other groups as expected. The Work Programme is not working as the Department intended and flaws in contracts have led to unnecessary costs. The Work Programme has the potential to achieve value for money. The Department has recognised that to do so it needs to make changes to contracts, improve information on performance and reduce unnecessary payments.

Figure 21
Summary assessment of the Work Programme

The Work Programme has performed better against previous welfare-to-work programmes than it has against the Department's intentions

		Previous programmes		Department plans or intentions
Performance				
Easier to help (job outcomes)	~	Similar performance (paragraph 11)	✗	Improvement not achieved (paragraph 12)
Easier to help (sustainment)	~	Similar performance (paragraph 11)	✗	Improvement not achieved (paragraph 11)
Easier to help (off benefit)	✓	Higher than previous (paragraph 14)	✓	Higher than expected (paragraph 14)
Harder to help (all outcomes)	~	Similar performance (paragraph 16)	✗	Improvement not achieved (paragraph 16)
Services				
Targeting support	n/a	No previous committments	✗	Lower than intended (paragraph 17)
Monitoring of minimum services	n/a	No past minimum service standards	✗/~	Monitoring initially ineffective (paragraph 18)
Costs				
Overall costs	✓	Lower costs and risk transfer (paragraph 19)	~	Costs driven by performance (paragraph 19)
Valid payments	✓/~	Improvements in overall control environment (paragraph 21)	✗	Invalid sustainment payments (paragraph 22)
Performance management (incentives)	n/a	No past incentive payments	✗	Incentive payments for all (paragraph 23)
Performance management (termination)	n/a	No performance based termination	✗/~	Only break clauses (paragraph 24)
Contract management	✓/~	Dedicated provider assurance and monitoring teams (Figure 11)	✓/~	Multiple changes to avoid costs (paragraph 25)

Notes

1 In some cases we have interpreted Department intentions, or based our assessment on a reasonable view of what the Department would have intended. For example we assume that the Department would intend to pay only for valid outcomes.

2 Improvements in control environment identified in past reports.

Source: National Audit Office assessment of Work Programme performance

Appendix Two

Our evidence base

1 We completed our review of the Work Programme after analysing evidence we collected between January and April 2014.

2 **We reviewed the Work Programme against its original aims.**

- We reviewed the business case and other documents to understand the programme's priorities.
- We carried out semi-structured interviews with officials to gather further information on how the programme was developed and managed.

3 **We reviewed operational performance.**

- We analysed the Department's management information on referrals, attachments and job outcomes and made comparisons to previous employment programmes.
- We requested performance data from each of the 18 Work Programme contractors and received responses from 17 contractors. We also asked contractors about the challenges they face that may affect operational performance.
- We reviewed the documentation supporting the Department's decision to terminate one of the contracts held by Newcastle College Group. We also interviewed senior management from Newcastle College Group.

4 **We reviewed the performance management regime.**

- We reviewed documentation and guidance on the performance management regime to understand the requirements placed on contractors.
- We reviewed the Department's data on performance against the contractors' minimum performance standards and against generic performance criteria.
- We interviewed and ran group discussions with performance managers and compliance officers to find out more about the monthly monitoring processes and how contractors are held to account against their contracts.

5 We reviewed the Department's control of costs.

- We visited five contractors as part of the financial audit validation of systems and controls for attachment, job outcome and sustainment payments.
- We requested cost data from each of the 18 contractors including a breakdown of forecast and actual programme costs, and details of payment arrangements for subcontractors.
- We reviewed departmental documents about contract changes and the associated costs savings these changes were expected to attract.

Appendix Three

Performance comparisons explained

1 In this Appendix we describe some of the limitations of our comparisons with welfare-to-work programmes, including:

- major differences between programmes;
- differences between compared cohorts and payment groups; and
- possible impacts of limitations on comparisons.

Comparisons for easier-to-help groups

2 We compare Work Programme easier-to-help performance with Flexible New Deal and New Deal 25 Plus (**Figure 22**). Flexible New Deal is a more recent programme and only ran for a short period, so may be more similar to the early stages of the Work Programme. New Deal 25 Plus lasted longer and may be a better indicator of a mature programme.

3 The programmes defined payment groups and performance differently. **Figure 23** on page 52 shows which groups and measures we considered, and explains some of the differences in the timing and measurement of cohort performance.

4 Because the programmes are not perfectly comparable we consider some of the possible impacts of differences on measured performance compared with Flexible New Deal (**Figure 24** on page 53). Some factors suggest the Work Programme is performing well relative to Flexible New Deal or dealing with more difficult conditions. Other factors work in the opposite direction. We comment on the possible direction of these impacts, but in many cases cannot assess the extent of the impact. Where possible we have already adjusted for differences in the estimates we use in our report.

Figure 22

Overview of the Work Programme, Flexible New Deal and New Deal 25 Plus

Our comparison programmes have different outcome definitions and payment breakdowns

	Work Programme[1,2]	Flexible New Deal[2,3]	New Deal 25 Plus
Period of scheme	2011–2016 (referrals) 2013–2020 (payments)	October 2009 – May 2011 (referrals)	1998–2010 (referrals)
Number of participants	1.6 million (expected)	404,000	825,000 individuals had 1.3 million spells
Cost of scheme[4]	£2.4 billion (expected) £1,500 per referral	Terminated early £1,590 per referral (expected)	Not available
Length of programme for a participant (planned)	2 years	1 year	Up to 10 months Three stages of 3 or 4 months
Outcome definition	6 months sustained work including interruptions, defined as 26 weeks with employment in the time since attachment (up to 30 months)	26 weeks in employment within a 30 week period	No outcomes Scheme aimed for job entries
Payment breakdown	20 per cent attachment 25 per cent outcomes (payment-by-results) 55 per cent sustainment (payment-by-results)	40 per cent service fee 60 per cent outcomes (payment-by-results)	Largely Jobcentre Plus with the latter stages including payment-by-results

Notes

1 Work Programme referrals and costs are based on Jobseeker's Allowance payment groups using Departmental estimates from May 2014.

2 Both Work Programme and Flexible New Deal use payment-by-results so the costs per referral of each programme vary with performance.

3 Flexible New Deal was cancelled early and its cost per referral is based on the Department's estimate in the Work Programme business case.

4 Costs relate to payments to contractors; they do not include benefit savings or wider impacts of employment.

Source: National Audit Office analysis of departmental documents and modelling estimates

Figure 23

Payment groups and cohorts for easier-to-help comparisons

Our comparison programmes have some differences in outcome definition

	Work Programme	Flexible New Deal	New Deal 25 Plus
Participant groups	9 payment groups including Jobseeker's Allowance and Employment and Support Allowance claimants	Jobseeker's Allowance claimants	Jobseeker's Allowance claimants aged 25 and over
Base for comparison	Payment group 2 Jobseeker's Allowance claimants aged 25 and over	Payment group 1 and 2	Payment group 2
Claimant mix	Includes some lone parents		
Length of programme for a participant (actual)	Variable cohort duration, with 10 cohorts completing 2 years (up to March 2014)	9 cohorts completed 1 year participation. 11 cohorts were participating when the programme was terminated	As planned
Outcome definition	6 months sustained work including interruptions, defined as 26 weeks with employment in the time since attachment (up to 30 months)	26 weeks in employment within a 30 week period	No outcomes Scheme aimed to achieve job entries

Source: National Audit Office summary of Department for Work & Pensions' documents

Figure 24

Impact of comparisons between Flexible New Deal and the Work Programme

Design differences between programmes can impact on comparable performance

	Description	Possible impact on measured performance of the Work Programme relative to Flexible New Deal
Design differences		
Length of programme	Work Programme lasts 2 years compared to 1 year for Flexible New Deal. Work Programme also measures outcomes over a longer period	Increases relative performance (In our report we adjust the performance measure for Flexible New Deal to account for this difference)[1]
Breaks in employment	Work Programme measures cumulative employment and allows interruptions, while Flexible New Deal measured continuous employment	Increases relative performance (In our report we adjust the performance measure for Flexible New Deal to account for this difference)[2]
Validation regime	Work Programme job outcome claims must pass an off-benefit check (which cannot be appealed), and an in-work sample test which excludes around 7 per cent of claims. On Flexible New Deal the off-benefit check could be appealed and there was no in-work test	Decreases relative performance (because Flexible New Deal is overstated) (In our report we adjust the performance measure for Flexible New Deal to account for this difference)[3]
Economic conditions		
Benefit history of participants	On average people spent more time on benefit before joining the Work Programme than Flexible New Deal[4]	Decreases relative performance
Job opportunities available	Both programmes ran in difficult economic conditions. Conditions for the Work Programme have improved recently	Unclear impact on relative performance in early stages of programmes; likely to increase recent performance[5]
Logistical differences		
Capacity of contractors	Work Programme referrals were initially much higher than contractors had planned for and are now much lower than expected. The Department expects contractors to cope with volume changes, but contractors have cited difficulties[6]	Decreases relative performance for early cohorts, and increases relative performance for more recent cohorts
Establishing operations	Work Programme introduced quickly and contractors were still establishing operations in the early months	Decreases relative performance for early cohorts

Notes

1 Length of programme adjustment: Flexible New Deal measured outcomes within 18 months of referral (18 per cent) whereas Work Programme measures up to 30 months after referral. Based on the experience of the Work Programme over later months, we adjusted Flexible New Deal performance upwards based our estimate of how it might have performed over a similar period.

2 Continuous employment adjustment: Unaudited information from contractors suggests up to a third of job entries are achieved by participants that have already had one period of employment. We used Departmental estimates to adjust Flexible New Deal performance upwards to account for differences.

3 Validation adjustment: We have decreased the performance of Flexible New Deal by 7 per cent to allow for the differences between the programmes' validation regimes.

4 In the four years before referral, the first participants referred to the Work Programme spent 118 weeks on benefit (57 per cent of their time). The first participants referred to Flexible New Deal spent 97 weeks on benefit (47 per cent).

5 Performance on the Work Programme has periods of rapid improvement for all contracts, in all payment groups, which suggests external conditions affecting performance have improved. The Centre for Economic and Social Inclusion calculate that the performance of early cohorts was lowered by difficult economic conditions. In the long term, the Department's analysis of the non-intervention rate (the proportion of participants that would achieve employment without any assistance) suggested that economic conditions do not affect performance significantly. Neither Flexible New Deal, nor the Work Programme, had a method to assess the current proportion of outcomes achieved above the level that would have occurred without a programme.

6 Referrals of Jobseekers Allowance claimants in the first year of the Work Programme were 37 per cent (172,000) higher than anticipated. Referrals in 2013-14 were 28 per cent (100,000) lower than original forecasts.

Source: National Audit Office summary of the Department for Work & Pensions' documents

Comparisons for harder-to-help groups

5 We compare Work Programme harder-to-help performance with Pathways to Work (**Figure 25**). The different programmes defined payment groups and performance differently. **Figure 26** shows which groups and measures we considered, and explains some of the differences in the timing and measurement of cohort performance.

6 Because the programmes are not perfectly comparable we consider some of the possible impacts of differences on measured performance (**Figure 27** on page 56). Some factors suggest the Work Programme is performing well relative to Pathways to Work or dealing with more difficult conditions. Other factors work in the opposite direction.

Figure 25

Overview of the Work Programme and Pathways to Work

Participants sustained employment at a similar level to the Department's estimate of previous programmes

	Work Programme[1]	Pathways to Work
Period of scheme	2011–2016 (referrals) 2013–2020 (payments)	2008–2011 (referrals)[2]
Number of participants	416,000 (expected)	564,000 individuals had 588,000 spells
Cost of scheme	£363 million (expected) £870 per referral	£600 per referral
Length of programme for a participant (planned)	2 years	Five interviews spaced 4 weeks apart with no formal end date
Outcome definition	6 months sustained work including interruptions, defined as 26 weeks with employment in the time since attachment (up to 30 months)	No outcomes. Scheme aimed to achieve job entries
Payment breakdown	Expected breakdown: 20 per cent attachment fee 25 per cent outcomes (payment-by-results) 55 per cent sustainment (payment-by-results)	Intended breakdown: 30 per cent service fee 70 per cent for job starts (payment-by-results) (Extra service fees to cope with cashflow problems were awarded to most contractors)

Notes

1 Work Programme referrals and costs are based on Employment and Support Allowance payment groups using Departmental estimates from May 2014.

2 Provider led Pathways was 'rolled out' in two phases. The first phase began in December 2007, and the second in April 2008. Each covered approximately 30 per cent of Great Britain.

Source: National Audit Office summary of the Department for Work & Pensions' documents

Figure 26

Payment groups and cohorts within programmes

Our comparison programmes have different payment groups and measurements of performance

	Work Programme	Pathways to Work
Participant groups	9 payment groups including Jobseeker's Allowance and Employment and Support Allowance claimants	Incapacity Benefit claimants
Base for comparison	Payment group 6	Payment group 6
Claimant mix	Employment and Support Allowance Claimants with 3 and 6 month prognoses Employment and Support Allowance claimants with 12 month prognoses from November 2012	All Incapacity Benefit claimants with mandatory referrals to provider-led services
Length of programme for a participant (actual)	Variable cohort duration, with 9 cohorts completing 2 years (up to March 2014)	As planned
Outcome definition	3 months sustained work including interruptions, defined as 13 weeks in the time since attachment (up to 27 months)	No job outcomes measured, only job entries

Source: National Audit Office summary of Department for Work & Pensions' documents

Figure 27

Impact of comparisons between the Work Programme and Pathways to Work

	Description	Possible impact on Work Programme relative to Pathways to work
Design differences		
Length of programme	Work Programme measures outcomes over a longer period than Pathways	Increases relative performance
Breaks in employment	Work Programme measures outcomes allowing 3 months of employment in multiple spells. Pathways only measured job entries; Departmental analysis suggest 88 per cent lasted 3 months or longer	Undetermined impact on relative performance. The Department does not have complete job entry data
Validation regime	On the Work Programme, the Department accepts claims that pass an off-benefit check (which cannot be appealed), and an 'in-work' check which excludes 7 per cent of claims	Decreases relative performance (because Pathways to Work performance is outdated)
Economic differences		
Benefit history of participants	Jobseeker's Allowance participants spent more time on benefit before joining the Work Programme than similar participants on previous programmes, but this data is not available for Employment and Support Allowance claimants	Unclear impact on relative performance
Case mix of Employment and Support Allowance	All Incapacity Benefit claimants were referred to Pathways to Work. Until November 2012, Employment and Support Allowance claimants with a 12 month prognosis were not referred to the Work Programme	Increases relative performance of cohorts referred before November 2012
Job opportunities	Pathways to Work operated in different economic conditions. Circumstances for the Work Programme have improved recently. The extent to which this affects performance is unclear	Unclear impact on relative performance
Logistical differences		
Referral rates	Initially, Work Programme referrals were much lower than contractors had planned for and a limited proportion of all referrals Referrals are now higher than expected and are a significant proportion of all referrals so contractors have to focus on performance	Decreases relative performance for early cohorts, and increases relative performance for more recent cohorts
Establishing operations	Work Programme introduced quickly and contractors were still establishing operations in the early months	Decreases relative performance for early cohorts

Source: National Audit Office summary of Department for Work & Pensions' documents

Appendix Four

Comparison with Universal Credit and Personal Independence Payment

Figure 28
Comparison of major programmes

The Work Programme is a more mature programme than other Department programmes we have reviewed recently

	Universal Credit[1,2]	Personal Independence Payment[3]	Work Programme
Summary description			
Aims	Simplifying benefits and encouraging people to work	Better targeting of support for disabled claimants	Helping the long term unemployed and harder to help into work
Description	Replaces six working-age benefit streams with a single payment	Replaces Disability Living Allowance for people aged 16 to 64 years old	Replaces several previous welfare-to-work schemes
Implementation timetable	2013–2017	2013–2017	2011–2017
Claims received	2,000	166,000	1.5 million (referrals)
Claimants expected by 2018	8 million	3.6 million	2.5 million (referrals)
Current stage	Pathfinder extension and developing new long-term plans	National roll-out of new claims and partial roll-out of reassessments	Full running of the programme
Programme management			
Timetable	April 2013 pathfinder and October 2013 new claims, compared with internal assessment of start date in April 2015	April 2013 controlled start and June 2013 national new claims roll-out. Reassessments planned between October 2013 and October 2017	May 2011 controlled start followed by full running from June. Referrals end in 2015 but support for existing participants goes on until 2017
Management approach	Agile adopted up to early 2013 then changed to more traditional method	Agile used throughout the design and implementation	n/a
Clarity of end state	Repeated concerns over clarity of end state and attempts to redefine blueprint	Clearly defined end state identified early in programme development	Clear objectives with high degree of uncertainty over baseline performance and deadweight

Figure 28 *continued*

Comparison of major programmes

	Universal Credit[1,2]	Personal Independence Payment[3]	Work Programme
Programme management *continued*			
Transparency and challenge	Good news culture and fortress mentality identified through third party reviews	No issues reported as part of third party reviews	Regular performance data published
Financial control of suppliers	PricewaterhouseCoopers identified serious failings of financial control	No major failings identified by PricewaterhouseCoopers	No extrapolation of errors in sustainment payments
Departmental oversight	Large programme board with frequent changes in attendance; lack of challenge	Programme board with a consistent membership that met regularly	High degree of performance management of contractors
Assurance reviews	In mid-2012 failure to address recommendations from assurance reviews	Majority of recommendations accepted and steps taken to address these	Evaluation ongoing
Restructuring	Major simplification exercise in early 2012, followed by restructuring in autumn 2012	Limited narrowing of scope for online claims and internal systems	Next phase of welfare to work support being considered

Notes

1 The description of Universal Credit reflects the position in September 2013 when the National Audit Office last reported on its progress. The Department has been working to address concerns raised since May 2013.

2 Universal Credit claimants expected reflects the Department's plans from December 2012.

3 The description of the Personal Independence Payment reflects the position in February 2014 when the National Audit Office reported on its progress.

Source: Comptroller and Auditor General, *Personal Independence Payment: early progress*, Session 2013-14, HC 1070, National Audit Office, February 2014

Made in the USA
Monee, IL
05 November 2026

67383063R00038